How to Build a Great Food Relief Project

The 10 Ingredients of Success

By Paul Rodney Turner

International Director of Food for Life Global

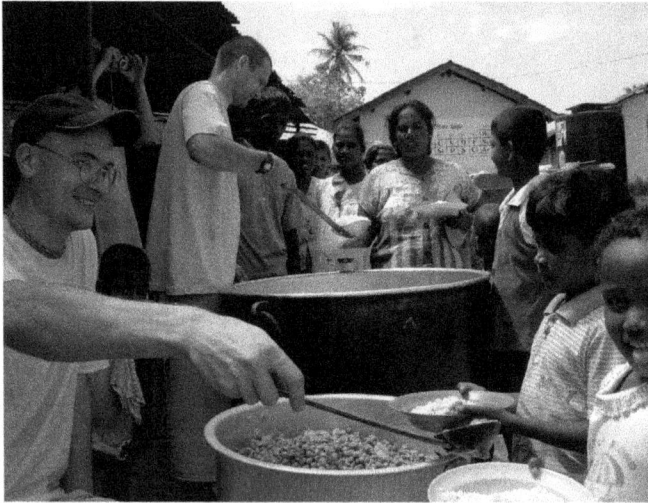

First published in 1996, as a booklet for Food for Life volunteers titled, *"The 10 Ingredients for a Successful Food for Life Program."*

Revised and updated for people of all faiths.

Contents

Acknowledgements

The first person I need to thank is my spiritual preceptor, A.C. Bhaktivedanta Swami Prabhupada, who introduced me to India's Vedic culture of hospitality and inspired the modern-day Food for Life program.

Following his example, Mukunda Goswami, my predecessor as director of Food for Life, guided my first steps to share the joy of prasadam with the world. I am not sure how I could have survived without his encouragement all these years.

Thanks must also go to Stephen Covey, who inspired me to create a formula for success that could be shared with our affiliates. His *7 Habits* model became my *10 ingredients*.

Finally, thanks to Nancy Adams for her editorial contributions and for understanding what I wanted to convey to the reader.

Preface

Defining your goals

If you wish to bake a cake, you first envision the type of cake you want—the flavor, color, consistency, topping, etc.— and then you go about collecting the appropriate ingredients to create that particular cake. Similarly, if you wish to develop a successful charitable feeding program, you must have a clear vision of the goal(s) you wish to achieve with your humanitarian service. In other words, what is your vision? Do you want to see more meals distributed to the needy in your city? Do you want to see the leaders of society becoming model examples of health and vitality? Maybe your goal is introduce more nutritious meals in your local school?

Whatever your goal(s), they should all be formulated into a concise **Mission Statement**, which will then become the focus for all your charitable efforts.

Systems—the recipe

Every successful person, organization, and project started out with a well thought-out, systematic plan and a clear vision of the future. In every sphere of life we see systems. There are systems for management, development, law enforcement, maintenance, and even destruction. Mother Nature is a dynamic and elaborate eco-system.

If you wish to see the successful execution of your charitable mission, you will need to adhere to some form of system. Your system should lend itself to variation; be sensitive to time, place, and circumstance; and allow for innovation. Your system should be based on principles or essential ingredients that will ensure the success of your "recipe" or formula.

The following system contains 10 essential ingredients for building a successful food relief program, which are formulated to suit the needs of an international palate.

We emphasize here that all 10 parts are **essential**, just as all the ingredients within a delicate cake recipe are essential, although some are more important than others. It may well be that your charitable program already incorporates some of these ingredients. However, we strongly recommend that you collect **all 10 ingredients,** and if necessary, begin remaking your charitable feeding program until it is the finest in town!

Paul R. Turner

International Director

Food for Life Global

www.ffl.org

Introduction

Since the early years of my career with Food for Life it has been my passion to share the meaning of hospitality, as it is understood in Vedic culture.

One of the key teachings of the Vedas is that all sentient beings are essentially equal in spiritual quality and thus intimately connected through a beautiful symbiotic web of service. Essentially, we are all one big family, seemingly separated by race, gender and species, but in reality, inseparable and interdependent.

With this understanding, I felt the need to expand the scope of the Food for Life charity, from an outreach program of ISKCON[1] to a social change movement that anyone could embrace and participate in.

The result of that quest is this condensed instructional booklet that can serve to empower you and your friends, church, or community group to start your very own feeding program based on the same principles that govern every Food for Life program. It is my hope that your project will one day become an affiliate of the founding charity.

Swami Prabhupada, the inspiration behind ISKCON's Food for Life project, passed away in 1977, but the instructions he left to all Food for Life volunteers were crystal clear: "Everyone should get a chance to take prasadam[2]." He also stated: "(T)his activity should be expanded universally to stop sinful eating habits as well as other behavior befitting only demons." He obviously knew the power of transformation that prasadam could have on society, and thus, right from the very beginning of his work in the United States, he encouraged the preparation and distribution of sanctified food to the public.

As I meditated on these mandates, it became more and more obvious to me that fulfilling them was far beyond the capacity of one charitable organization, but in truth required a more expansive and dynamic approach—an approach that would demand openness, love and faith.

---

[1] ISKCON – The International Society for Krishna Consciousness.

[2] Sanctified plant-based food that has been offered to God in devotion.

I realized that at the heart of these instructions was the need for people to understand the concept of "prasadam" and its capacity to elevate consciousness. "We simply have to share this knowledge and let go," I thought. This belief led me to write a book, *FOOD YOGA - Nourishing Body, Mind & Soul*™, to teach people how to make food an essential part of their daily spiritual practice, and then to write this companion booklet, which focuses more on the practical execution of pure food distribution to the public for those outside the Krishna tradition.

In truth, however, this booklet is an updated and revised version of the one I wrote for Krishna Food for Life volunteers in 1996. The subject matter has been expanded, but the essential message remains the same, and the ingredients I share for my formula of success are as they were back then with only minor modifications.

Finally, I feel the need to stress the absolute necessity that any project wishing to affiliate with Food for Life Global must serve only plant-based foods. The reasons for this mandate are many, foremost of which is that there is no justification for taking the life of an innocent animal for food. Such cruelty flies in the face of the Food for Life philosophy—that all living beings are created equal and should be respected as such. I have shared some additional reasons in a later chapter.

Moreover, no new project will be recognized as an affiliate of Food for Life Global unless it complies with our *ahimsa* policy in relation to food production, selection, preparation, and serving.

On behalf of Food for Life Global volunteers around the world, I thank you for your sincere desire to make a positive difference in the world and join us in this noble vision.

Summary of the 10 Ingredients

1) UNITED VISION

United we stand, but divided we fall. You must build a committed and unified team by creating a *Mission Statement*. All members must be on the same page, both philosophically and emotionally convinced. Establish internal and external goals.

2) FIVE ESSENTIAL STRATEGIES

- Identify and target the social weak points. (Find the need.)
- Feed children and students (the future).
- Network with other organizations. (Get connected.)
- Do not exclude anyone. (Reach the masses.)
- Feed your friends and family. (You need their emotional support.)

3) EXCELLENCE

Quality is more important than quantity. Although selfless service is not *of* this world, we are living *in* the world. Strive for excellence in service, food quality, vehicles, uniforms, and etiquette. Be thoroughly professional.

4) INVOLVE PEOPLE

Everyone can serve in some capacity. Be open-minded. Utilize your members. Start a supporters' club. Interest. Inform. Involve.

5) PROPAGATE, PROPAGATE, PROPAGATE!

Propagating selfless service to humanity is the best way to create unity and peace in the world. Promote your program everywhere—on vehicles, uniforms, promotional materials, newsletters, merchandise, and the Internet. Develop relationships with the media.

6) ENDORSEMENTS

Third party endorsements, especially from opinion leaders, are your ace cards to wide-scale success. Use all forms of media, including newspaper, radio, and television, as well as letters from celebrities and dignitaries and verbal praise.

7) SOCIAL INTEGRATION

Become part of the community and be seen as relevant. Holidays and festivals are terrific opportunities. Celebrate Christmas, Hanukah, Kwanza, Janmastami, Ramadan, Mother's Day, Father's Day, Easter, New Year, etc; attend festivals and fairs of all cultures; distribute meals at sporting events, public park beautification days, school fairs, and government health initiatives; attend charity meetings; write to the newspaper and offer opinions on social issues. Be willing to share your facilities and donate your time, skills, and meals.

8) TRUTHFULNESS

It is stated in the ancient scriptures of India, "Truthfulness is the last leg of religion." How is your organization demonstrating truthfulness? Truthfulness attracts money! All charities should be above suspicion and demonstrate accountability with an open-book policy. Strictly adhere to ethical fundraising policies.

9) PATIENCE AND "FRIEND-RAISING"

Fund-raising begins with friend-raising. You must sell your dream (Vision) to your donors as an investment in a mission. But before asking for help, become *qualified* by answering three important questions (explained later). Remember the 80/20 principle: 80% of your income will come from 20% of your donors. A newsletter is an essential tool in your fundraising toolkit, as are direct mail, letter writing skills, and the ability to research and apply for government and corporate grants.

10) PURITY—THE FOUNDATION

Always remember how interdependent we are. Never become proud, for purity, humility, and love are the most powerful forces in the universe.

THE BASICS

Before we get into the essential ingredients of a successful food relief program, we need to address the basics of setting up an organization. Basically, there are two ways you can do this:

1) Register a new non-profit organization with its own tax ID number and corporate officers.

2) Cooperate with an established non-profit organization. (This approach is also discussed in a later chapter on strategy.) Even though it is strategically important to expand one's own service by cooperating with other reputable organizations, it is still necessary to establish at least some form of organization, even if you just create a website, business stationery, and a bank account.

Let's focus, therefore, on the more involved process of creating your very own non-profit organization. I will not go into explicit details here, since there are many other books available that deal with this subject, but here are the steps in a nutshell:

a) **Choose a name for your organization**. Research trademarks and business names at USPTO.gov and your local government office first.

b) **Get incorporation application forms** at your local government office, or file online with a service like bizfilings.com. You will need to list the aims and objectives of your organization, and you can use the guidelines provided by Food for Life Global or standard templates provided by local government for this purpose.

c) **Find two other enthusiastic and reliable people** to join you in forming a corporate board consisting of a president, secretary, and treasurer.

d) **Hire or find a volunteer CPA or bookkeeper** to manage your finances.

e) Once you are incorporated and your organization has an Employer Identification Number (EIN), file **with the IRS to get tax exempt status**. Your CPA will typically do this for you.

f) **Set up a business bank account** with two people as signers for checks (usually treasurer and president).

g) **Set up a PayPal account** or some other merchant service, and associate your charity bank account with it.

h) Now that you've taken care of the legal and financial tasks, it is time to **set up a website and create business cards**. Your website can be as simple as a few pages outlining your mission, services, and how people can contact you with questions or to volunteer or donate.

i) **Create an e-newsletter** and a way for people to subscribe on your website.

j) **Keep donors and volunteers informed** of your progress, and never stop appreciating them.

These are the basics. If you'd like more in-depth information, check your local library or bookstore for books on incorporation.

Let's now look at the key ingredients that make a food relief or any charitable service stand out from the crowd and be successful. Here are the 10 ingredients of success...

1) UNITED VISION

United we stand; divided we fall

Every successful team requires the united interests and beliefs of every member, from top to bottom, inside and outside the organization. Or in some cases, one inspired person's dream will be shared and adopted by others. There is always a team behind every successful person, be it a football player, horse trainer, boxer, politician, salesman, or spiritualist.

None of us live in a vacuum. Every person, at some point in life, requires the help of another. So whether the team builds the vision together or adopts one individual's vision, there is no question that a *team* is what makes a dream happen. In other words, it is not a team of champions that wins, but a *champion team*.

Commitment to the dream (Vision)

Stephen Covey, author of *7 Habits of Highly Effective People*, and master of personal and corporate management, declares that commitment to the mission of the organization only happens when people are *practically involved*. **"No involvement, no commitment,"** he writes. "Note it down," he adds. Covey later expands on this message when he introduces the principle of *synergy:* the art of valuing the differences, or the understanding that the sum of the whole is greater than the sum of the individual parts. "We should see how individuality can complement the team," he explains. With this in mind, be open to the opinions and perceptions of all our members, both inside and outside the team. You must create forums for expression, where all members can give input and feel valued. Ideally, you should involve all members in **creating the mission statement,** thereby charging it with relevance, potency and realism. By doing so, you will harness firm commitment on all levels.

Building your support team

The way to build your support team is to sell a dream! Every human being hankers for a purpose in life, an expression, or a way to leave a legacy. The Indian philosopher Chanakya Pundit once wrote: "Because the world is temporary, one should try to do something immortal." The purport is clear, but Swami Prabhupada, founder of Food for Life, gave this message a spiritual charge by explaining that the *only* truly immortal thing to do is to serve Krishna[3] (God).

The beauty of Food for Life, behind its seemingly exclusive concern with worldly matters, is a spiritual activity called *prasada seva*[4]—the sacred act of distributing pure plant-based food. Therefore, what appears to be an ordinary welfare activity is actually a completely wholesome way to nourish the body and soul with sanctified plant-based food. This is explained in detail in my book, *FOOD YOGA – Nourishing Body, Mind & Soul* ™.

Monitoring the pulse

Managing an organization is in many ways like monitoring your health. When the doctor puts his finger on your pulse, he immediately understands something about the health of your heart.

Similarly, by regularly listening to the opinions and feelings of your team (inside and outside the organization), you will be able to maintain good organizational health, with clear channels of communication and expectation. Asking your donors, supporters, and team members to complete periodic surveys is a great way to do that. Find out what they are thinking, what they like or dislike about your management. Hear their solutions to your problems. Involve them in decision making, planning, and formulating strategies. Always ask questions and hear people out. There is no loss, but only immense gain to be made, for a truly wise man knows how to take gold from a dirty place.

Three questions to ask your team

Creating a mission statement for your food relief project can be a stimulating and creative experience. To facilitate the free flow of thought and creativity, arrange to meet with your team away from the work place,

---

[3] *Krishna* is a name of the Supreme Personality of Godhead. It literally means the "All Attractive One" and is used by millions of Hindus throughout the world in their daily prayers. God has many names, of which *Krishna* is one.

[4] *Prasada* literally means "mercy," and in the case of Food for Life, it means food that has been sanctified after first offering to God. For information on offering food, see section *Making an Offering. Seva* means "Service."

in a quiet area, free from disturbance. Sitting in a circle, ask the following questions, allowing time for team members to write their answers:

i) Who are we?

In as few words as possible, try to come to some consensus on exactly who you (the team) believe you are and why your project is important to you and society. The last thing you want is an identity crisis or complete ambiguity.

ii) How do we want to be perceived?

What image or impression do you want to convey to the public? Identify obstacles that stand in the way of this perception.

iii) What do we want to achieve?

Be specific here. Don't be afraid to think big, but don't just throw out big ideas; instead, attach them to people and time frames. (Identify *who*, *what*, *when*, *where,* and *how*.) The response to this question will represent your team's **internal goals**, which are even more important than the external goals.

Next, have each person read his or her answer to the group. There should be no criticism, only sharing and appreciating each person's viewpoint and concerns. Write the essence of each answer (a short sentence or one word) on a board so that everyone can see. After everyone has been heard, discuss the points raised, and then try as a group to formulate a response that best reflects the group's opinion, keeping in mind that the goal is unity in diversity.

Do the same for each question, summarizing on paper the three answers and other points brought up in the discussion. Hand out a copy to each person and ask them to meditate on the questions and answers until you meet again in a week.

Mission statement

Next it is time to formulate your mission statement, encapsulating every member's needs, concerns, and desires (both inside and outside the organization). It should be as concise as possible, but filled with meaning and drive! Now, reread, redefine, and edit the statement again and again until you arrive at something you are all totally satisfied with. (This phase may take a few weeks and many meetings.) Ideally, it should be contained in one sentence. **The mission statement should become your internal constitution**, the driver for every decision or activity to be carried out by your team. Your mission statement must be flexible, and you should review it regularly to make sure your team is aligned with it. Don't just file it away! Post it on the wall in large, bold lettering, and print it on the back of business cards so that it can be internalized and carried by all the members.

Discussions on pure food

The ancient teaching of the *Vedas*[5] and most other bona fide scriptures agree that spiritual purification can be achieved by first purifying the tongue. *"Hallowed be Thy Name"* is the first of seven petitions in the Lord's Prayer in the Bible. In the Hindu traditions, chanting God's name is considered the *Yuga dharma*, or the primary spiritual activity for the present age, and thus, much emphasis is given to the chanting of the *Maha Mantra*. The same Vedic scriptures explain that praising God is the medicine and eating *prasadam*[6] is the diet for curing the ills of materialism. Therefore, it may be worthwhile to set aside time to discuss the spiritual benefits of pure food distribution.

A good source for such discussion is the *Bhagavad-gita*, which can be obtained from any ISKCON temple. Because these activities are fundamental to all spiritual traditions, one can adapt them to the practices of one's own preferred spiritual path.

The main points are to acknowledge the necessity of purifying the meal before it is distributed to the public and to construct a practical program that can be adopted by all members of the team. More about the purification process will be discussed in the chapter "Making Offerings."

---

[5] Ancient scriptures originating in India and used by Hindus throughout the world.

[6] Pure plant-based food literally meaning "mercy" and in the context of this document it refers to food that has been sanctified through a process of offering to God.

Philosophically convinced

Like any socially conscious activity, your mission must have a strong and persuasive philosophical basis so that all volunteers will remain enthusiastic and determined. We therefore offer the following philosophical points in support of a project like Food for Life:

i) Spirituality begins with the tongue

According to the *Vedas*, it is stated:

> Translation: "No one can understand the transcendental nature of God with materially contaminated senses. Only when one becomes spiritually purified beginning with engaging the tongue in tasting sanctified foods are the transcendental qualities of the Lord revealed."

Spiritual purification begins with engaging the tongue in spiritual activities, of which eating sanctified food is paramount. Who can argue this universal truth—that God is beyond the ability of our mundane senses to perceive? Therefore, we need a process of personal purification to qualify us to perceive the divine presence of God.

ii) A solution for world peace

Swami Prabhupada once stated: "Simply by liberal distribution of *prasadam* and *sankirtana*[7] the whole world can become peaceful and prosperous." The reasoning behind this statement is simple: food speaks all languages. In its purest form, food has the ability to unite, to heal, and to pacify. Food that is devoid of negative energy associated with the suffering of animals and that has also been prepared with loving intention has the power to transform hearts, which can lead to true and lasting peace.

iii) Medicine and diet

According to the ancient medical science of India, *Ayurveda*, curing a disease requires the correct prescription of medicine and diet. To

---

[7] Group chanting of mantras, typically consisting of names of God.

administer one without the other is practically useless. Swami Prabhupada often explained that prayer can be likened to medicine, and eating sanctified food is the proper diet for curing the disease of materialistic consciousness.

iv) A plant-based diet is good for the planet

In 2006, the U.N. Food and Agriculture Organization (FAO) produced a report on global warming that clearly identified factory farming and livestock as the number one cause of environmental damage. Global warming poses one of the most serious worldwide environmental threats in human history. Yet by focusing entirely on carbon dioxide emissions, major environmental organizations have failed to address published data showing that other gases are the main culprits behind global warming. As a result, they have neglected to adopt what might be the most effective strategy for reducing global warming in our lifetimes: advocating a vegetarian diet.

By far the most threatening non-CO_2 greenhouse gas is methane, and **the number one source of methane worldwide is animal agriculture.** Methane is responsible for nearly as much global warming as all other non-CO_2 greenhouse gases put together—**21 times more powerful than CO_2.**

v) A plant-based diet is good for health

Three studies published in the *Journal of the American Medical Association* prove a link between a plant-based diet and a reduced risk of cancer. The studies not only show that high consumption of fruits and vegetables wards off a variety of cancers, but also that consuming red meat multiplies the risk of colon cancer.

The studies found that a plant-based diet prevents cancer and enhances health at many different levels, including cardiovascular health. Dr. T. Colin Campbell, Professor Emeritus of Cornell University and author of the groundbreaking *The China Study*, is regarded by many as having produced the definitive epidemiological examination of the relationship between diet and disease, or more specifically, between cancer and animal protein.

Registration & your external goals

You'll need to register your food relief project with the appropriate government department(s), who can give you templates to use as a guideline and revise as necessary in developing your articles of incorporation. Likewise, you can start with the list below as your guideline, use as written or edit to suit, and add your program's own unique set of aims and objectives. (NOTE: If you wish to affiliate with Food for Life Global, it is imperative that adopt aims and objectives that are complimentary to Food for Life Global and that your articles of incorporation clearly state that you will adhere to the guidance of Food for Life Global.)

The aims and objectives of a typical Food for Life Affiliate are as follows:

In pursuance of the mission of Food for Life Global Inc., the organization aims to act as an affiliate project under the authority and guidance of Food for Life Global Inc. and will have following aims and objectives:

a) To provide nutritious plant-based meals to the public, without discrimination and wherever necessary, within the state of registration.

b) To teach the effectiveness of a plant-based diet in improving physical and mental health, protecting the environment, and creating peace and prosperity;

c) To promote the benefits of a plant-based diet through books, pamphlets, video, public discourse, and cooking lessons;

d) To counsel disadvantaged people with the aim of improving their quality of life through abstention from intoxicants; meat, fish or eggs; gambling; and all other forms of immoral activity.

e) To assist in fulfilling the mission of Food for Life, that everyone should get a chance to eat pure plant-based food.

f) To conduct retreats for disadvantaged youth and to provide training programs to build their self-esteem and improve their life skills.

Once you have registered your program, you will need to apply for tax-exempt status by completing and filing a standard form with the taxation department (IRS in the U.S.). We recommend that you consult a good lawyer to advise you in registering your charity and applying for tax-exempt status. You cannot afford to make a mistake.

MOTTO #1: *Build a champion team.*

2) FIVE ESSENTIAL STRATEGIES

The following five strategies are the most effective ways to develop your food relief program. You may be able to accomplish more than one strategy with just one well thought-out program; the greater number of these strategies you can incorporate into your project, the more effective your project will be. Each strategy has an important part to play in firmly establishing your project.

1. Target the Social Weak Point

Identify and target the social need (homeless people, single mothers, the elderly, refugees, AIDS victims, veterans)

Try to identify the social need in your city by researching government reports; talking to other charity organizations, the police, and people in the community; and reading local newspapers. You may find one or all of the above examples.

Identify the weak point and target it with a solution that is in line with your core activity – food distribution. Your solution should be relevant and sensitive to the needs of both the community and the people you're trying to help.

For example, if there is an unemployment problem, you could approach the government for a grant to employ people to grow vegetables for your project. It is simply a matter of being creative and learning to connect every situation to your agenda, or seeing every issue as an opportunity to expand and promote your project.

2. Feed the Children

Feed children and students (university clubs, school breakfast clubs, orphanages, homeless shelters, hostels)

Feeding children and students is the most important of all strategies, simply because children and students are the future of society. Every government and society invests a major portion of its wealth, time, and energy in its children and students. Targeting or helping these groups is a sure way to receive support and respect from the community.

The Food for Life Mid Day Meal Program in India is a classic example of this. Thousands of schools across India receive fresh, hot vegan/vegetarian meals from Food for Life daily. The project has received numerous accolades in the media and continues to grow in size daily.

A more humble approach would be to start a student breakfast club at your local school to serve those children who come to school without having had a nutritious breakfast. Another is to start a Food for Life club on campus.

The first goal in organizing a Food for Life (FFL) campus chapter is to find a few individuals to form a core group—individuals who are energetic and committed to the formation of the FFL chapter on their campus. This committed group of activists will do the lion's share of the work, drive the organization, and ultimately determine the chapter's success or failure.

Trying to start a chapter by oneself can be very overwhelming. Creating a core group is a great way to distribute the work and the rewards of organizing a new Food for Life chapter.

How to organize the chapter

Advertise to the student body your intention of starting an FFL chapter to see if there is any preliminary interest. Advertise through e-mail, flyers, the campus newspaper, or any other media you can access. Be persistent.

If there is interest, plan a meeting to discuss what you envision your chapter will do and what others want the club to do. Use resources from animal rights and vegan groups, such as FARM (www.farmusa.org) and Compassion Over Killing (www.cok.net).

Once your group is established, discuss when you would like to meet, how much time you can realistically dedicate to this chapter, what events you would like to do, and how you will create enthusiasm for your cause on campus. These are not always easy things to do, so start small, be flexible, and be sure to use resources of local Food for Life staff as well as the past experiences of other Food for Life campus chapters.

3. Partner with other organizations

The Red Cross, Salvation Army, police, Adventists, United Nations, OXFAM, *Save the Children*, vegetarian/vegan societies, animal rights organizations, Greenpeace, community supported agriculture (CSA), etc. have all, at some time, assisted or worked with a Food for Life project somewhere in the world. This strategy is not only logistically sound, but it will also serve to build your reputation with the greater community, create opportunities by connecting you with the right people at the right time, and help you gain access to the necessary funds, skills, and facilities you need to help build your charity.

There is no need to reinvent the wheel. Everything your food relief project needs (skills, land, money, facilities, people, buildings, etc.) is already available. You simply have to access these facilities by partnering with the right people. Because food is such a fundamental need, your program will offer a wonderful opportunity for such cooperation.

There is no disputing the value and efficacy of giving people healthy food – it's a universally accepted principle. When you make the effort to network, a host of facilities, skills, connections and opportunities will open up before your eyes.

4. Do not discriminate

Provide pure plant-based food for everyone else (i.e., snack foods, festivals, shops and offices).

"Everyone is spiritually poor," stated Swami Prabhupada; therefore, "by feeding everyone, automatically you feed the poor."

No one should miss out on the experience of *prasadam*. Developing pure food snacks for mass distribution, then, is an important component of this strategy. These snacks can be sold to shops and offices, or distributed for free at meetings, gatherings, and conferences. You can also use these snack foods to advertise your charity by printing information on the packaging.

The main point behind this strategy is to understand that ultimately we all need good food, and whether it is in the form of a healthy snack bar or a full meal, no one should be denied.

Food for Life, in that sense, is not just a feeding program for the poor, but more of a nutrition education service, or social change movement (using food as its medium) that also provides meals to the poor. Again, no one should ever be denied a meal. Never discriminate, rich or poor.

5. Charity begins at home

Feed the family (i.e., congregation, friends, and spiritual festivals).

It's important to convince your friends, family, and congregation about the need for and value of a plant-based food program.

One of the most common problems a program director faces is not having enough qualified people involved in the program, either because people just don't get it or because their priorities are off. To remedy this, hold education seminars to inspire your core group and dispel misunderstandings. Most importantly, feed them! There is nothing like education through sensual experience.

It is also essential to realize that sharing pure food is central to the development of loving relationships. Your volunteers, therefore, should seek opportunities to serve pure plant-based meals to their core public, and thus win their love and support. Hospitality is an important part of any spiritual tradition, and we all know that charity begins at home.

Finally, everyone likes a festival! At least 50% of any festival's success depends upon the quality and presentation of the food served. Therefore, seek every opportunity for your team to participate in festivals, especially those your congregations are sure to attend, as this is a sure way to win people over and diffuse enemies. Offer to provide the food, or at the very least, be the team that serves the feast!

MOTTO #2: *Be a soldier and a diplomat on the battlefield.*

3) EXCELLENCE

Quality is more important than quantity

When it comes to food, nothing is as important as the quality or excellence of the ingredients, preparation, and presentation. Food for Life's founder wanted volunteers to strive towards perfection. He was never satisfied with second best or mediocrity. "God will not accept the grandest offering from a dirty kitchen, but He will accept the humblest offering from a clean kitchen," he said. When it comes to preparing food, there is nothing as important as cleanliness. The success of the spiritualization of the food depends on it.

Our loving intention is demonstrated through the cleanliness of everyone involved in the food production, including those who grow the food, harvest the food, transport the food, buy the food, prepare the food, and serve the food. Serving food is equally as important as cooking, because serving, too, has a direct bearing on the satisfaction of those being served.

Volunteers should be trained to serve respectfully, selflessly, and with enthusiasm. The condition of the food transportation vehicle will also affect the public's appreciation and acceptance of the charity. Vehicles should be spotlessly clean and look like they belong to a professional organization.

Business Logic

According to the latest business logic, the idea of quality over quantity fits like a square peg in a round hole in today's corporate environment. The reason is simple – businesses are established to make money as quickly as possible and at the highest possible margins. Therefore, crafting high quality products can be expensive and time consuming. They also must be sold at much higher, less attractive prices to the average consumer in order to make them profitable. Whereas, lower quality workmanship, manufactured speedily in outsourced factories with a minimal time commitment per product, are typically far more profitable, with higher margins and lower, more attractive price points. Look no further than the likes of Wal-Mart and Target who use this model.

However, when it comes to the non-profit industry, quality is critically important. With all the scams and bad press from non-profit executives taking million dollar salaries and operation budgets of up to 90% in some cases, public faith has been shattered.

If you want to build credibility in this industry, you have to focus on quality, which means not only being selective in the ingredients you use to prepare the meals and the standards of cooking, but also in the overall operations of the charity, from accounting to volunteer coordination.

Living in the world

The modern world largely operates on a superficial platform. Image, packaging, name, dress, hairstyle, jewelry, and transport all have their influence on the public's perception of an organization or individual. Although we may not, in a spiritual sense, be *of* this world, we are undoubtedly living *in* this world, and therefore, it behooves us to abide by the codes of conduct accepted by the society in which we live and work. Your group needs to present itself as a respectable organization with members that act with integrity.

Uniforms are also essential to a good public image. Volunteers should dress immaculately. "First dress, than address," should be our motto, and we should always strive for *excellence*.

MOTTO #3: *Do everything with loving intention.*

4) INVOLVE PEOPLE

Everyone can serve

Abraham Lincoln, once said, "To ease another's heartache is to forget one's own." The fact is service is like food for the soul. We all feel inspired and happiest when we are serving others and making them happy. This is true for every person on the planet and therefore, as a public service organization, it is your duty to provide service opportunities. "There are two ways of spreading light - to be the candle or the mirror that reflects it," Said, Edith Wharton. In other words, we can be a facilitator of service or a cheerleader to inspire more.

Volunteers are the heart and soul of any non-profit, so be open-minded, and try to give as many people as possible a chance to get involved in your project. A food relief project is certainly capable of engaging a wide variety of people in service, be it sponsoring, donating cash or kind, fund-raising, delivering, packing, cleaning, cutting, or distribution. In all circumstances, however, everyone should be trained to meet the standards and policies of the organization.

The people in your group, congregation, friends, and family will obviously be your best initial resource for support and service. Therefore, use the community notice board and newsletter to inform them, interest them, and ultimately involve them in your food relief service. Do whatever is necessary to acknowledge those people who have made a commitment to support the organization or who are presently serving in some practical way. For a religious congregation, the worship service is a good time to remind people, report progress, and get new commitments. You may also try to have special worship service lectures.

Home gatherings are also excellent for building teams and maintaining enthusiasm. Visit your congregation regularly and get them to hold their own charity support group gatherings. Meetups are another good way to build a team. Every project begins in seed form by talking about it. Another key to building an enthusiastic team is to get people speaking with others about their experience, realizations, and ideas.

Ways to Inspire Volunteers

Source: http://topnonprofits.com/

1. Thank your volunteers and thank them again. Show appreciation in varied ways and always mention volunteers who make your organizational successful.

2. Reward your volunteers. Volunteers have many motivations. While they are supportive of your mission, making connections, being seen at your events, and becoming more immersed in the experiences of your staff and constituents are all perks with appeal. Remember that some individuals volunteer to have more contact with others in event and social settings. Some of your most dedicated volunteers may be easing back into work-related settings after retirement, the loss of spouse, as grandchildren have left for college. Get to know your volunteers and what excites them about what you do.

3. Provide an experience connected to your cause. Nurture engagement—not just tasks needed by your organization. The stories of those whose lives are enriched or changed by your nonprofit's work will inspire your volunteers.

4. Create a community or team from your volunteers base. Connecting your volunteers and maintaining open communication channels among your staff and volunteers help to build community. In person thanks and feedback events are the best ways to fuel connection between volunteer work opportunities. These can be supported by electronic (such as discussion forums) and feedback tools (like surveys) but there's nothing like thanking volunteers with a party or just picking up the phone.

5. Share your volunteers' success stories to demonstrate the importance difference they make. Showcase your volunteers and how their time and talent contribute to your organization's growth.

6. Honor top volunteers in both big and small ways. Small recognition efforts mean a lot. Volunteers understand that the constituents receiving your programs and services are top priorities. But those donating their time and assistance will appreciate being recognized by name in print, online, and in event settings. A token or certificate for volunteer service is always a nice touch. Consider designating a "Volunteer of the Month" recognition or something that occasionally features volunteers in your newsletter, social media, and other outlets.

7. Cultivate your volunteers for bigger roles. Your volunteers may also be leaders — staff, advisors, board members, and consultants. Your volunteer pool may yield not only other human resources, but donors. Sure you'll have volunteers who just want to show up and assist with whatever task you provide. However, care and feeding of all of your volunteers is critical for your organization's reputation and growth.

8. Grow your volunteer pool through recruitment of volunteers by...your volunteers! Word of mouth is great advertising. Your volunteers are likely your best recruitment asset. Provide ways for volunteers to invite others to join them. Gather information about the best way to reach the contacts of your volunteers and provide information in what ever medium is more easily shared by members of your volunteer pool.

Think about who volunteers with your organization. Know them well enough to make the best assignments and to provide the perks that will make your volunteers keep coming back–and telling others about your mission and the roles they play in your success.

Supporters Club

There may be people who do not have the time to practically involve themselves in your food relief program, but who would still like to participate in a meaningful way. Give them a chance to do so by establishing a supporters club for the purpose of expanding distribution and furthering the aims of your charity. Get participants working on fundraising drives, pure food business ventures, promotional materials, media events, and training programs. No one should be denied the opportunity to serve the charity. Be creative and open-armed.

MOTTO #4: *Be broad-minded and compassionate.*

5) PROMOTE YOUR BRAND

"As bold as brass..."

So the saying goes, to illustrate how confident and bold one must be while on duty. All volunteers should be enthused to tell the world about the amazing activities of the charity and specifically the founding charity, Food for Life Global. What other organization currently serves up to 2 million meals daily to the needy? What other organization promotes a holistic approach to the health and wellbeing of humans, animals, and the environment? Indeed, Food for Life has raised the bar in public service. Therefore, every person who uses a Food for Life affiliate logo on their uniform should be conscious of the responsibility that goes along with it: to represent an organization that was not only founded on integrity, but also has the most far-reaching positive agenda in the world.

Since the first impression is often the lasting impression, managers must take care to ensure that every volunteer is trained in what to say, how to act, and how to dress to project a good impression of our organization. *Everything a volunteer does communicates a message.*

Your charity name everywhere!

In terms of marketing, the very least we can do is to have good signage on all vehicles, if only just a small magnetic sign with the project logo and URL attached to the door can help to educate thousands about your charity.

To project a professional image, it is also essential for volunteers to wear uniforms (aprons are best, but jackets and t-shirts are also good). Promotional materials help to educate the public and the media, and a newsletter is necessary for the church congregation and your donors.

A minimum of two volunteers should work full-time on developing media relations through personal visits, food giveaways, and flyer distribution. One or more volunteers should attend charity meetings and conferences and network with directors of other organizations, celebrities, opinion leaders, and prominent government officials.

Production and sales of charity merchandise is a great way to involve people on a practical level. This merchandise can be used for fundraising, as gifts for donors, or maybe as free advertisements. Finally, the Internet offers a golden opportunity to impact a large audience with the least expenditure. Promote the program on your blog and various social media sites like Facebook and Twitter. NOTE: All public relations initiatives mentioning Food for Life Global must be pre-authorized by Food for Life Global.

Corporate Sponsorship

It is estimate that corporations in the US spend over $20 billion dollars a year on corporate sponsorship. Wouldn't you like to get just a piece of that money?

If you do, the first thing is to be clear about your demographic and your platform. The following notes are from Linda Hollander, the founder of the Women's Small Business Expo.

Your platform is your message and your fan base--people who know you or who align themselves with people you know. Your demographic is the market you're after, and you want to have statistics about that market at your fingertips. For example, if your market is women, be aware that they make or influence 85 percent of purchasing decisions, and that they are starting businesses at twice the rate of men.

Find out the spending power and purchasing habits of your target market. Research the median income and educational level.

Consider the publications your demographic reads. Then ask for media kits from those publications. According to Hollander, media kits will reveal amazing things about your demographic--all provided for free.

Don't forget cause-related marketing, either. "This is so hot that it's scorching. People want to purchase from companies that give back to the community. If you change lives in a positive way, that's cause-related marketing." Sponsors will be eager to come aboard, Hollander says.

Have a great sponsor proposal. "Without it, don't even bother," Hollander advises. "It has to be completely compelling." The person you show that proposal to has to show it to accounting to get approval and a check. You need to connect personally with your champion in the company.

In addition, be aware that there's a certain format for how the proposal has to look, Hollander says. "It has to have certain language and certain sections."

36

Start with a story. It could be your story, or the story of someone whose life you changed. "Whatever you do, tell a story. This will get your proposal to stand out and make an emotional connection." Hollander points out that there's a person in the company you approach who's going to make a decision about sponsoring you. "That person has to make an emotional decision to give you the money," she says.

Describe what you do. This is your mission statement. It explains why you do what you do. You also have to have really great benefits for the sponsor you're approaching.

Describe your demographics.

Create an advisory board. "If you don't have experience, surround yourself with people who have experience. Show potential sponsors that you have an A team."

Ask for the money. "They don't call you to ask how much money you want," Hollander says. "A sponsor once said to me, 'If I don't see a menu of prices, I throw it out.'

Hollander offers a training class that includes her proposal template, and she personally reviews each student's proposal. "If you don't have me look over your sponsor proposal, have someone who has done it look it over," she says. "Otherwise, you're going to be wasting your time and it's going to be an exercise in frustration."

Promise deliverables. Don't just promise media coverage. Promise specific media coverage: "I will give you media coverage in the hometown business journal. It has a circulation of 60,000 people making more than $100,000 a year."

Don't sell yourself short. Ask for $10,000 to $100,000 from each sponsor. "I see people asking for $1,000. That's not going to cut it. You're dealing with a well-paid person in a corporation. It's not worth their time if you're asking for $500 or $1,000."

Hollander also advises asking for a year-long program, not just a single event. "Make it a whole year, because then you don't have to keep going to the well."

Find the right person to approach in the company. "Ask for the marketing department. That's the best place to start," Hollander says. She noted, however, that in some companies, the appropriate department might be public relations, community affairs, public affairs, supplier diversity or brand management.

Whenever possible, Hollander advises, introduce yourself by telephone, not e-mail. "This is a relationship business," she says. "You have conversations; you don't just e-mail back and forth." Besides, a lot of corporations have good firewalls, and your e-mail may not get through. **"E-mail once you have the relationship,"** Hollander says.

Try to avoid filling out an online form. That's a screening device, she says. "It's like the black hole on Star Trek where something goes in and never comes out."

Be impeccable with your word. When you're courting a sponsor, always do what you say. Sponsors will test you. If you can't get information, tell them why. Always be on time or early for an appointment. Let them know you are a person of integrity. "You get one chance to make an impression, and if you burn the bridge, you can't go back."

Always follow up. "So many people lose deals because they don't follow up," Hollander says.

Be brief, be brilliant and be gone. Ask for what you want, but don't take up a lot of a potential sponsors' time doing it.

You can't help anybody until you help yourself. Until you're financially secure and strong, you can't help all the people you want to help. Corporate sponsorships are a way to make you strong and give you the resources you need, Hollander says. They also add to your credibility. She also advises that you publicize your corporate sponsors on your website to let people know you are playing at a higher level in business.

The Food for Life logo

If your intention is to become a bona fide affiliate of Food for Life Global, the official Food for Life Affiliate logo must be used in all circumstances. The files can be purchased from Food for Life Global. Any adjustments or additions to the logo or standard marketing materials must be approved by Food for Life Global.

MOTTO #5: *Be bold, but sensitive.*

6) ENDORSEMENTS

All forms of media—newspapers, radio, television, Internet, and letters from celebrities and dignitaries—are valuable methods of endorsement that you can use to build the reputation of your charity and help establish its acceptance in society. "It's not what you know, but whom you know," is an often-quoted saying that clearly illustrates the power of endorsement. Endorsements are one of the building blocks of a good reputation, and a good reputation is the hallmark of successful non-profits. Therefore, a practical strategy must be employed to get opinion leaders, businesses, or other non-profits to endorse your project.

Newspaper articles or television reports are equal to tens of thousands of dollars in positive advertisement! Praise from opinion leaders has equal merit because they have the power to motivate the masses.

"Whatever action a great man does, common men follow. And whatever standards he sets by exemplary acts, all the world pursues." - Bhagavad-Gita.

Your ace cards

As noted in the *Gita*, endorsements by influential people are your ace cards to gaining the wider support of the public and the keys to opening the doors of opportunity. These endorsements should be used and not packed away in the archives. Moreover, they should be available for other FFL affiliates to use when the need arises. You should think of the world first and your project second and in this way help to solidify the global unity of FFL affiliates.

The Internet has created a global village. What happens in one part of the world is now relevant to and often impacts other parts of the world. You therefore need to view your project as a member of a global family of similar non-profits, and demonstrate this connection in practice.

MOTTO #6: *It is not what you know, but WHOM you know.*

7) SOCIAL INTEGRATION

Removing negative association

Generally speaking, ISKCON, the organization behind the founding of Food for Life, is not seen as an organization of social contributors. However, most people are also unaware that the few monks they may interact with on the street represent only a small fraction of the ISKCON membership.

Most members of ISKCON are responsible citizens with families and tax-paying jobs. Nonetheless, some potential supporters may balk at supporting you because of this historical association. It is, therefore, very important to explain that your project, like all bona-fide Food for Life projects, is completely non-sectarian and an independent of any religious institution. Even Food for Life Global is non-sectarian and independently incorporated from a religious institution.

What practical things can we do, then, to avoid or counteract misunderstandings and bogus labeling?

Holidays and festivals—a terrific opportunity!

Observing social holidays and festivals such as Christmas, Hanukah, Kwanza, Ramadan, Mother's Day, Father's Day, New Year, etc., is one practical and powerful way to change public opinion. The effort can also lead to forming innovative partnerships and educating the public about the other aims and objectives of the charity. Every festival or holiday culminates in a feast, and so every festival or holiday offers an opportunity for pure food distribution. We should seek these opportunities because they demonstrate for all to see that your volunteers are not only socially conscious and responsible people but also open minded and non-sectarian.

Attending festivals and fairs; distributing pure food at sporting events; participating in public park beatification days, school functions, and Government health initiatives; attending social welfare meetings; writing to newspapers offering opinions on social issues; sharing facilities; and donating time, skills and pure food to other organizations—these are all ways to show that you and your team are meaningful, socially concerned, and active and proud members of the community. People who are tuned in to the needs of society as sensitive, compassionate, fun-loving and normal human beings.

Let's cite an example: Food for Life volunteers in Russia often have to deal with the conservative and biased views of the Orthodox Church and the media, who basically adhere to the unfriendly paradigms explained previously. Never did they expect that Food for Life volunteers would celebrate Christmas and a variety of other social festivals, and when they witnessed it, the experience drastically changed their viewpoint.

On one occasion, the Moscow Food for Life team baked a two-ton cake for the famous Russian Children's Day festival. The huge cake in the form of a swan caught everyone's attention with its colorful decorations and Food for Life banner. "*Now we know you are good people*," reported one newspaper. The thousands of children and parents who received a piece of that stunning cake quickly threw away all contention and misunderstanding. Similarly, "God bless you Food for Life" was the praise heard on Christmas day, when the same volunteers prepared a pure feast for a local orphanage in Moscow.

Christmas is traditionally a family day, and so feeding orphans was a thoughtful and intelligent strategy. It quickly erased all negative thoughts and left a positive impression of the volunteers as compassionate, socially concerned, and responsible people.

MOTTO #7: *YOU must build the bridge.*

8) TRUTHFULNESS

Truthfulness is Godliness

In an age of increasing decadence, purity—like truthfulness —stands out like sunbeams on a dark and rainy day. Practically speaking, little truthfulness remains in the modern world. Even in everyday business, where profit must be made to survive, the realization of profit all too often means that someone or some company was cheated.

Your volunteers should be the epitome of honesty and trust, above suspicion. According the *Vedas*, Truthfulness is an austerity of speech and a quality of the noblest members of society. Unfortunately, in the modern age, many people are involved in some form of cheating just to survive. Swami Prabhupada would often say that there are only two classes of people: the *cheaters* and the *cheated*. However, for reasons stated above, we can see that most people belong to both. Considering this, just imagine how much your members will stand out in the crowd if they are impeccably truthful, and how much trust your organization will gain if you can establish a solid reputation of honesty.

How do we demonstrate truthfulness?

Showing accountability by opening the organization's account book is one practical step towards this end. Practicing what we preach and doing what we say we are going to do is another. Strict fund-raising policies must be enforced to deter all forms of illegal collecting in the name of your charity or Food for Life.

Today, nearly all charitable organizations encounter some problems with abuse, and therefore, as an organization representing the pure ideals of Food for Life Global, you should not allow a few ill-motivated individuals to spoil the reputation of the whole organization. It only requires one person.

Truthfulness attracts money

Some people contend that cheating is necessary in order to make ends meet or get ahead in this fast-paced, competitive world. We strongly disagree, and the founder of Food for Life clearly stated: "God is the husband of the Goddess of fortune. He can give us the world, but we are not ready." History shows that where there is an exceptional level of truthfulness, money and support for flourish.

Take for example the case of David Dobson, Food for Life director in Philadelphia. Very early on in the development of his project, Mr. Dobson received a substantial grant from the state government. By good management and financing, Mr. Dobson was able to finish this approved project while using only half of the funds allotted to him. Unlike most people, Mr. Dobson decided to send the remaining cash back to the government department explaining to them that he had met his goals. You can just imagine the look on the government officer's face when he opened up that envelope containing a check for the unused money! "Who are you people?" he asked Mr. Dobson on the phone. "No one ever returns money."

Without a second thought, Mr. Dobson had seemingly thrown away a lot of money, but in doing so he demonstrated an uncommonly high level of integrity and professionalism, thereby depositing a huge sum of TRUST in the government's emotional bank account. The following years saw Mr. Dobson receiving million-dollar grants, and today he has tens of millions of dollars in government contracts! There could be no clearer example of how, by being truthful, one can collect more money than most volunteers could ever dream of.

MOTTO #8: *Live by truth and become empowered.*

9) PATIENCE AND "FRIEND-RAISING"

Selling the dream (Vision)

Fundraising, in essence, means friend raising. Simply put, if you want money, you must make friends. Or, if you're struggling because you do not have enough money, analyze your methods of cultivation. Are you making friends, or are you begging?

Most people detest the "We're in danger of collapsing" approach or the "Help, it's an emergency!" appeal. Because such efforts are overused, they can bore potential donors and, in time, even make them bitter. A more positive and constructive approach is to offer your donors service opportunities—a mission—or to sell them your project's dream. Remember: **If you want to build a team (supporters), you have to sell the dream (your vision).** Unfortunately, many non-profits struggle to survive, simply because members are not patient enough to invest the necessary time, energy, and money in the service. They're after the quick-fix.

80/20 Principle

Like a universal truth, we see the 80/20 principle everywhere within business and personal life. Within the context of fundraising, it simply means that 80% of your income will come from only 20% of your donors. What this means in a practical sense is that although all donors need to be recognized, you must give extra attention to that 20% of donors. Typically, it is within this 20% that you will also find your opinion leaders within the community, and such leaders will influence others.

Becoming qualified to ask

We have purposely placed this topic as number nine in the list for a very good reason: until you have added the above ingredients to your program, you are not going to be in a solid position to ask for funds. At this point, your team's vision should be clear; you should be targeting needs in the community and have earned a reputation for quality and consistency. You must be well known and endorsed by the "right" people—people who matter to those you're asking for money. Your program should be well integrated with the community; something your donors can be proud of supporting and connecting with. But above all, *you must be truthful* to the point that the public would never question your fundraisers. Of course, getting to this level, or being able to gather all these ingredients, is not going to be easy. But the point is, the more of these ingredients you have, the more success you'll have when you ask for support (cash or kind).

Three important questions

Following are three basic questions most people or companies consider before committing to a donation, along with hints as to how you can answer their questions:

> **1) Is this organization doing something valuable? Are they feeding the right people and fulfilling a genuine need in the community?**
>
> **HINT**: Research and target the weak points. Do a program for young people, especially school children or students. Promote this information widely. Work with reputable people and organizations.
>
> **2) Are these people accountable? Do they have a reputation for honesty, integrity, and accountability? Will they spend my money properly, in the way they say they will?**
>
> **HINT**: Produce a newsletter for the donors, showing accounts and giving the names of donors. Make a good reputation one of your principal goals, and devise strategies to achieve it. When you spend donations, send a letter and report to those donors. Never do something contrary to what you promise. Always spend the money (donations) exactly as the donor expects (as you promised or planned). Always *under-promise and over-perform*.
>
> **3) What is the behavior of these people like? Do they practice what they preach? Are they consistent?**
>
> **HINT**: Involve your donors in your project. Provide opportunities for them to serve food at your distribution spot

and attend your charity promotional events. Arrange to visit donors at their homes. Show them videos of your program, news reports and endorsements. Train your volunteers to deal with the public respectfully. Pay attention to the way volunteers dress and their etiquette in public. Remember: Every volunteer is under the spotlight. *Everything a member of the organization does is communicating a message.*

For further information on fundraising, we recommend you join your local chapter of fundraising professionals.

MOTTO #9 : *Your success is only limited by your imagination and your reputation.*

10) PURITY—THE FOUNDATION

Your personal health

When we speak of health, it must always include mind, body and spirit to be truly holistic. Of these three aspects, nothing is as important as your spiritual health, of which prayer or meditation is essential. Many leaders use the excuse of their managerial responsibility to neglect the most important and essential responsibility—their **spiritual nourishment**. Without exception, everyone who does this eventually becomes emotionally weak and ineffective. We are, by nature, spirits inside a material machine, so to neglect the health of our essence is much like neglecting to feed the driver of a car. At a certain point in time, if not nourished, the driver will die and the car will cease to move.

The essential point here is this: if you want to feel empowered to drive your project to the highest levels of success, you absolutely must give time to your own personal spiritual nourishment. Whether that takes the form of daily prayer or meditation, you must accommodate this need.

It is important to understand that the fundamentals of a project like Food for Life are not of this world, but are operating at a much higher vibration than most philanthropic endeavors. We get our strength, enthusiasm, and determination, therefore, from that same vibration (channeled to us through prayer or meditation), and not from mundane knowledge, wealth, or trickery.

In the same way, if we neglect the health of our minds by subjecting them to negative vibrations, fuel our bodies with inferior foods, or do not set aside enough time for quality rest and recreation, we cannot expect to be operating optimally.

Therefore, no matter what you may think is important, **your spiritual nourishment, beginning with *prayer or meditation,* along with loving attention to your bodily and mental health, must become your number one priority.**

MOTTO #10: *Charity begins at home – nourish your mind, body and spirit.*

Why FFL Serves Only
Plant-based Meals

People often ask why Food for Life's food distribution program is strictly plant-based. The following points briefly summarize the virtually countless reasons for adopting a plant-based diet.

Health

A plant-based diet has been shown to lower the risk for many chronic diseases, such as obesity, coronary artery disease, high blood pressure, and diabetes, as well as cancer of the colon, breast, prostate, stomach, lung and esophagus. A plant-based diet can also ease symptoms of menopause and provide relief from several digestive ailments.

According to the U.S. Centers for Disease Control (CDC) 76 million people are affected by food-borne illness each year. Although it's possible for any food to be contaminated, the most frequent and severe cases of food-borne illness come from meat and other animal products.

Studies at Yale University and elsewhere have shown that anywhere from 5% to 30% of people diagnosed with Alzheimer's disease actually had Creutzfeldt-Jakob disease (CJD), the human form of bovine spongiform encephalopathy (BSE), commonly known as mad cow disease. While no smoking gun has yet been found to link Alzheimer's to mad cow disease, there is ample evidence that Alzheimer's, CJD and BSE are similar in their origins and in progression. Furthermore, according to Dr. Lawrence Broxmeyer of Med-America research, the risk of developing Alzheimer's is three times greater for meat eaters than for vegetarians.

Environment

The FAO report by the United Nations in 2006 stated unequivocally that factory farming of animals for meat production has a bigger impact on global warming than all the plains, trains, buses, and cars on the planet combined.

Raising animals for meat consumes massive quantities of water. According to the article "How Our Food Choices can Help Save the Environment," by Steve Boyan, PhD (www.earthsave.org), eliminating just one pound of beef from one's diet can save as much water as could be saved by forgoing showers entirely for six months!

Runoff from factory farms containing chemicals and animal waste—one of the greatest threats to water quality today—has polluted more than 173,000 miles of rivers and streams in the U.S. (Environmental Protection Agency).

World hunger

Meat production is an expensive and inefficient use of food resources. According to John Robbins in *Diet for a New America*, the grain required to feed livestock in America for one day is enough to provide every person on earth with two loaves of bread.

Spirituality

Switching to a plant-based diet is good for the soul as well as the body. In making the change, we forgo our selfish consumption of scarce resources in an effort to feed the world, and we condemn the cruel and inhumane practice of raising animals in abhorrent conditions to feed our taste for meat.

It's easy

Nothing could be simpler than fresh fruits and vegetables from the earth's bounty. And as we become more aware of the negative impacts a meat-based diet has on the environment, personal health, and world hunger, plant-based alternatives are becoming more visible and widely available in the marketplace. Even some fast-food restaurants now offer vegan and vegetarian menu items.

It's less expensive

Not only is a plant-based meal more nutritious, but it allows Food for Life to serve more children for less money. On average, a typical Food for Life meal consisting of rice, dhal and vegetable stew will cost around 0.30 cents. That means that every one hundred dollars donated, Food for Life can serve at least three hundred meals.

PURE FOOD

How to purify your meal

It is now time to learn the art of spiritualizing your food and taking your eating experience to the highest level.

The *Prasadarian* principles explained in *FOOD YOGA - Nourishing Body, Mind & Soul*™ provide a good introduction to the science and benefits of consuming higher vibrational foods. Before we get to the actual offering procedure, however, it is imperative to observe the following principles, which are essential to the preparation of pure food (prasadam).

Clean hands and work area – This is the most important principle. Nothing impure should be offered, and this necessitates having a clean working environment, clean body, and clean clothes. It is also recommended that you set aside a special offering plate just for this purpose – one that is not used by anyone else.

Use only food and ingredients that are free from meat, fish, eggs, animal byproducts, and pesticides. Avoid non-organic and GMO foods and anything that has been contaminated by the suffering of other animals.

A humble and devotional attitude – Refrain from tasting the food while preparing it. Reflect on the food as a blessing from Mother Earth; respect that blessing, and be happy.

The offering – You must prepare the meal primarily for the pleasure of God or the Goddess. Your personal enjoyment should be second to the pleasure of the higher powers. It is this kind of selflessness that should guide your devotion.

The Final stage of offering

In giving many talks on spiritual eating over the years, I came to understand that it was important for people to feel comfortable with the act of offering food, both within the context of their own spiritual traditions, and also in understanding the fundamentals of why we should even consider offering food in the first place. This led me to creating the *Universal Food Offering Invocation™* to guide people in the art and science of creating higher vibrational food.

With sincerity, purity, conscientiousness, gratitude, selflessness, nurturing, respect, loving acceptance, humility, and above all, devotion, use the following invocation to purify your food before you serve it.

Note that this invocation first sets the framework for the humble and devotional attitude by reminding us of our temporality and dependence on the grace of higher powers. I offer this invocation as a guideline to the final stage of the offering process. I recommend that you adjust this invocation to suit the specific tradition that you are accustomed to, although I believe that the invocation as presented here is universal enough to satisfy one and all.

It should be noted that a more in depth explanation of the *FOOD OFFERING MEDITATION™ appears in the companion book, FOOD YOGA - Nourishing Body, Mind & Soul™.*

THE FOOD OFFERING MEDITATION

I am Spirit

I am born with no possessions

I will leave this world with no possessions

I am neither the permanent owner nor ultimate controller of anything in this world

Everything that comes to me is a blessing of the Divine.

Since food is the most basic necessity of life, I therefore offer
this food with love back to the energetic source from which it came, in order to purify it.

In doing so, I acknowledge the Supreme Enjoyer, Supreme Creator, and the divine Feminine.

With love and sincerity I humbly ask:
"Please taste this food first."

Note

For more information on the subject of offering food, I encourage you to read the companion book, *FOOD YOGA - Nourishing Body, Mind & Soul* ™.

HOLY FOOD IN THE JUDEO-CHRISTIAN TRADITION

By Chaitanya dasa (Br.Aelred)

The preparation, offering, and consumption of food have a central role in the Judeo-Christian tradition, as in all other religious traditions. Central is the understanding that God has blessed the earth, that it may be able to produce, and that man may be blessed in the eating.

Let us look at a variety of Biblical references to "holy food."

There is a vital passage at the end of Chapter 1 of Genesis—the first reference to food in the Bible, and the first reference to the food that was given to Adam and Eve, our first parents:

God said, "See, I give you all the seed-bearing plants that are upon the whole earth, and all the trees with seed-bearing fruit; this shall be your food..."

One Catholic priest said to me recently, "Your commitment to a vegetarian diet is justified by reference to Scripture." He was, of course, referring to the verse above. It is very interesting (and disturbing) that Christians consistently overlook (ignore?) this passage, and choose to follow the less desirable diet given following the Great Flood—the diet that allowed meat eating. Whenever I raise this matter there is an awkward silence...then a flow of excuses!

In the Old Testament book of Leviticus, chapter 22, there is a lengthy passage on the subject of holy food:

Yahweh spoke to Moses; he said: "Speak to Aaron and his sons: let them be consecrated through the holy offerings of the sons of Israel...

"Any one of your descendants, in any generation, who in a state of uncleanness approaches the holy offerings consecrated to Yahweh by the sons of Israel, shall be outlawed from my presence...

"...At sunset he will be clean and may then eat holy things, for these are his foods...

"They (lay people) must not profane the holy offerings which the sons of Israel have set aside for Yahweh. To eat these would lay on them a fault demanding a sacrifice of reparation; for it is I, Yahweh, who have sanctified these offerings."

We obviously have a greater interest in the New Testament, especially as it has to do with "the best son of God," Jesus. As you will remember, Swami Prabhupada referred to Jesus in these words. In the New Testament we have two themes of central importance:

1.The sharing of food by believers or devotees. In Acts 2: 42-47 we read the following:

These (the early Christian community) remained faithful to the teaching of the apostles, to the brotherhood, to the breaking of bread and to the prayers.

The faithful all lived together and owned everything in common; they sold their goods and possessions and shared out the proceeds among themselves according to what each one needed.

They went as a body to the Temple every day but met in their houses for the breaking of bread; they shared their food gladly and generously; they praised God and were looked up to by everyone.

In his First Letter to the Corinthians, St. Paul writes:

Whatever you eat, whatever you drink, whatever you do at all, do it for the glory of God...

Later in the letter (Chapter 11), St. Paul deals at length with the whole subject of the eating of food. He is scathing in his criticism of the behavior of some, specifically because the eating of food is presented in the context of The Eucharist or the Lord's Supper. I will quote the whole passage, since, outside the Gospels themselves, it is the most important teaching on the subject of holy food.

The Lord's Supper

Now that I am on the subject of instructions, I cannot say that you have done well in holding meetings that do you more harm than good. In the first places, I hear that when you all come together as a community, there are separate factions among you, and I half believe it—since there must no doubt be separate groups among you, to distinguish those who are to be trusted. The point is, when you hold meetings, it is not the Lord's Supper that you are eating, since when the time comes to eat, everyone is in such a hurry to start his own supper that one person goes hungry while another is getting drunk. Surely you have homes for eating and drinking in? Surely have enough respect for the community of God not to make poor people embarrassed? What am I to say to you? Congratulate you? I cannot congratulate you on this.

For this is what I received from the Lord, and in turn passed on to you: that on the same night that he was betrayed, the Lord Jesus took some bread, and thanked God for it and broke it, and he said, 'This is my body, which is for you; do this as a memorial of me.' In the same way he took the cup after supper, and said, 'This cup is the new covenant in my blood. Whenever you drink it, do this as a memorial of me.' Until the Lord comes, there, every time you eat this bread and drink this cup, you are proclaiming his death, and so anyone who eats the bread of drinks the cup of the Lord unworthily will be behaving unworthily towards the body and blood of the Lord.

Everyone is to recollect himself before eating this bread and drinking this cup; because a person who eats and drinks without recognizing the Body is eating and drinking his own condemnation. In fact that is why many of you are weak and ill and some of you have died. If only we recollected ourselves, we should not be punished like that. But when the Lord does punish us like that, it is to correct us and stop us from being condemned with the world.

So to sum up, my dear brothers, when you meet for the meal, wait for one another. Anyone who is hungry should eat at home, and then your meeting will not bring your condemnation. The other matters I shall adjust when I come.

In conclusion, I would say that prasadam holds a central place in the Christian tradition, indeed with an added dimension. What I mean by "added dimension" is the following: in the Eucharist/Mass/Lord's Supper, not only are bread and wine offered to God, and so set apart from mundane use, but they actually continue to manifest the presence of Jesus Christ. Jesus Christ is actually present in every Mass; indeed, the bread and wine are arca vigraha (the worshippable form) of the Lord. Such is the Catholic and Orthodox doctrine of the Real Presence.

The Relationship Between Your Temple, Church or Community Group and Your Food Relief Program

On paper, register your food relief program as a separate legal entity from your church, so as to avoid conflicts with government and corporate policies on religious organizations and to position the program for the maximum support available from society and State.

The most successful Food for Life programs in the world are those that work within the church management structure; either through church volunteers and facilities or church funding (either directly or indirectly, as in the case of church seed funds or contributions from the congregation). The obvious question arises then: where do we draw the line on donations to the charity being used to support the church? The answer is: **The church is justified in using charity funds to the degree that the church supports your project** (by providing vehicles, premises, facilities, food, volunteers, etc.). Here we see the beauty of a synergistic relationship: by the church supporting your project, your charity can in turn support the church through reputation building, financial support (to help pay church bills), food donations, etc. It can be argued that the volunteers need feeding as well. If your food relief project receives donated equipment or facilities, there is no reason why the same equipment or facilities can't be used for church purposes, so long as the charity's purposes are fulfilled first.

Obviously the greatest contribution a Food for Life affiliate program can make to the church is to build a good reputation as an organization making positive social contributions. This alone is sufficient to warrant the church providing full support and use of its facility to your project (both practically and emotionally).

Final note

In conclusion, I want to make it clear that *How to Build a Great Food Relief* is a quick reference and guidebook, and therefore, I encourage further reading on the topics discussed. In particular, *FOOD YOGA - Nourishing Body, Mind & Soul* ™ as it offers a more thorough investigation into the art and science of nourishing the spirit through food.

Most of us are too busy to plow through huge manuals, and therefore we're always on the lookout for a quick-and-easy formula. This is exactly what you have here: *The ingredients of a success formula!* I wish you well.

About the Author

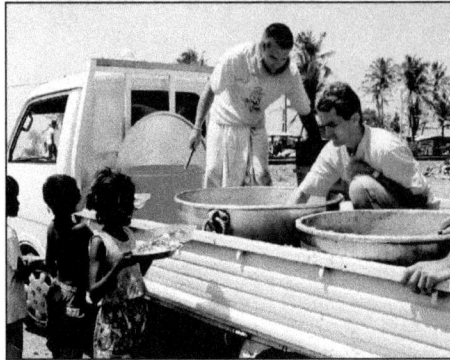

Paul Rodney Turner, also known as Priyavrata, a name given to him by his spiritual teachers, is the international director of Food for Life and the co-founder of Food for Life Global, the world headquarters for the charity.

Paul was born in Sydney, Australia in 1963 and grew up in the Western Suburbs of Sydney. At the age of 19, Paul left home to live a reclusive life in Sydney's Blue Mountains. Soon after he joined an ashram of similar spiritual seekers and took a vow of celibacy. For the next 14 years Paul, now known as Priyavrata das by his fellow Vaisnava monks, studied the ancient teachings of the Vedas as taught by His Divine Grace A.C. Bhaktivedanta Swami.

In the early years of Paul's life as a monk he learned vegetarian cooking and was soon cooking the Sunday feasts for the Sydney Hare Krishna temple, sometimes for as many as 300 guests. His desire to focus exclusively on India's Vedic culture of hospitality inspired him to start his own outreach project. At the time, Food for Life was a fledgling food relief organization with programs in Australia, USA, Western Europe and India.

Over the last 30 years, Paul has traveled to more than 65 countries throughout Europe, Asia, and the Americas, helping to inspire and set up new Food for Life projects and train volunteers. He also raised millions of dollars in funds; appeared on television and radio, and met with numerous government officials. In 1994, Paul wrote the official Food for Life training manual and in 1996 he wrote, sung and produced the first official FFL music CD called *Prasada Sevaya* (Service to holy food)

From 1999 to 2003 Paul was a Council Member and Magazine Editor for IVU (International Vegetarian Union), the official umbrella organization for vegetarianism worldwide. During Paul's travels he visited three war zones–Chechnya, Sarajevo and Sukhumi.

In 2005, Paul led an international team of volunteers to set up makeshift kitchens in villages across Sri Lanka in response to the Asian tsunami, where volunteers served freshly cooked vegetarian meals to tens of thousands.

In 2010, managed a team of volunteers to respond to the massive earthquake that hit Haiti. Over the next 6 months, tens of thousands of hot vegan meals were served to survivors. That same year, Paul also published a new edition of the Food for Life training manual.

In 2011, Paul published *FOOD YOGA – Nourishing Body, Mind & Soul*, an introduction to sacred path of becoming a *prasadarian* and learning to practice yoga to the highest standard. He also helped organize a team of volunteers to respond to the Tsunami disaster in Japan.

In 2014, Paul launched a numerology service, called The Number Advantage, www.numberadvantage.com

Along with directing Food for Life Global, Paul currently conducts FOOD YOGA workshops and retreats throughout the world and is working on several new book projects.

TWITTER: fflglobal

BLOG: www.paulrodneyturner.com

FOOD YOGA: www.FoodYogi.org

Support Food for Life Global

If you have enjoyed this booklet, please consider sending a donation to **Food for Life Global via www.FFL.org**. Your donation will be processed by our US Partner *A Well-Fed World* is tax-deductible. All donations will be used to further the aims of Food for Life Global, which are as follows:

- To provide plant-based meals to the disadvantaged, the malnourished, and victims of disaster (natural or man-made) wherever there is a need in the world.

- To establish Food for Life education centers throughout the world. These centers will provide free or inexpensive plant-based meals, counseling, yoga, and survival skills training.

- To establish Rural Academies for Youth (Food for Life R.A.Y. of Hope), whereby youth are trained in sustainable agriculture centered on spiritual values.

- To produce promotional and training materials for the development of Food for Life projects worldwide.

- To represent Food for Life to the government, media, and public through public lectures, newspaper articles, the Internet, and mail.

- To promote a food culture of hospitality based on spiritual equality.

- To raise funds on behalf of Food for Life projects worldwide, and to support them with small grants.

- To coordinate and sponsor emergency relief efforts conducted by Food for Life volunteers.

7 Habits of Highly Effective Food Distributors

Based on Dr. Stephen Covey's

7 Habits of Highly Effective People

1) *They are proactive:*

They don't see obstacles; they see God's hand in everything. They **smile** a lot while cooking.

2) *They begin with the end in mind:*

They envision and plan for the maximum amount of people to feed and the **maximum** impact on society. Their motto is: **quantity with quality** for the pleasure of God.

3) *They put first things first:*

Feeding the world is first! They are **selfless**, sense-controlled, and **hospitable**.

4) *They embrace an abundance mentality:*

They're convinced that there is enough *pure food* for everyone. **"Invite the world, we can feed them,"** they think. They're not misers.

5) They understand others:

They realize that **everyone needs pure food!** There is no need for philosophizing. "Let pure food do the talking," they say.

6) They are team players (synergy):

They are not autocrats, but cooperative, empathic servants of a united team. They realize that it is a **champion team** that succeeds, and not a team of champions.

7) They are balanced (mentally, physically and spiritually):

They are **equipoised,** knowing that **God is in control**. They are healthy, strong, and spiritually enlivened to do their best for a divine purpose.

Contact Food for Life Global

http://www.ffl.org

www.Facebook.com/foodforlifeglobal

contact@ffl.org

Ph: 202 407 9090